Patients' Cultural and Religious Issues

A guide for primary care

Patients' Cultural and Religious Issues

A guide for primary care

Sue Timmins

Education Business Manager
for the East Kent Community Training Alliance

Aeneas

First published in 2003
by Aeneas Press

PO Box 200
Chichester PO18 0YX
West Sussex
United Kingdom

Typeset in AGaramond
by Marie Doherty

Printed and bound by
Antony Rowe Ltd
Chippenham
Wiltshire
United Kingdom

ISBN : 1-902115-28-7

British Library Cataloging in Publication Data
A catalogue record of this book is available from the British Library

CONTENTS

ABOUT THIS GUIDE

People from different countries and cultures, and who follow religions other than Christianity, may have particular needs relating to the provision of health care. Every patient is entitled to a delivery of care which is sensitive to their needs, and which allows them to retain dignity. The Patient's Charter underlines this entitlement.

> 'The Patient's Charter and You' stated that '...patients can expect the NHS to respect (their) privacy, dignity, and religious and cultural beliefs at all times and in all places'.

The White Paper 'The New NHS: Modern, Dependable' subsequently stated the intention that everyone in the nation will have 'fair access to health services in relation to people's needs, irrespective of geography, class, ethnicity, age or sex.' It further stated the aim that the 'renewed NHS' will deliver 'a personal service which is sensitive and responsive to the needs of individual patients'.

It is therefore important that health care professionals have access to resources which will help them to increase their awareness of cultural and religious issues, and how this information may improve their delivery of care to their patients.

It is recognised that

> '... knowledge of a patient's culture can provide the health professional with some insight into the meaning of individual behaviour in illness, and improve the quality of care provided. Recognition by staff that a (patient) from a minority group may have different concepts about health and illness, as well as different expectations from consultations and care delivery, will go a long way in winning the confidence of the (patient), and ensure compliance with advice and treatment.'
>
> (Hopkins & Bahl, 1993)

In this guide, the term 'minority groups' is used to indicate cultural and racial groups who have their origins in countries other than the United Kingdom. These groups might therefore include, for example, Southern Irish, and the traveller population, as well as those people who may be identified more superficially by, for example, features or skin colour. Religious affinities apply both to people from immigrant stock and to those who may be described as 'white indigenous

British' who have by choice adopted faiths other than the State faith of Christianity.

In many rural parts of the United Kingdom, the host population is known to be in the majority; however, continuing numbers of people from elsewhere in the world enter the country, either settling by choice near their places of entry, moving to be near family groups, or relocating elsewhere under dispersal programmes. There are also many people from the host population who follow religions other than Christianity, either from birth or from personal choice.

In order to deliver appropriately sensitive services, health care professionals should be aware that patients from minority populations may have specific health care needs, either due to cultural or religious preferences, or because of recognised genetic predispositions to certain medical conditions.

Where there is a large minority population in one area, levels of awareness of these issues are usually relatively high. On the other hand, however, there are many rural areas where the perceived minority population is low in number, and consequently the need for awareness of issues relevant to these patients is not always seen as a priority. This can mean that, in certain areas of the country, health care continues to be delivered professionally, but may not always tailored to be sensitive to the needs of individual patients.

Recent research in primary care (Timmins, 2000) has revealed that, in rural areas, some GP practices have good levels of awareness of these specific needs, and an ability to meet them; however, the general level of awareness amongst those practices surveyed was relatively low. Many practices reported that they had not yet identified a need to provide culturally aware services, and some asked for help in developing this aspect of their work.

Many health care professionals working both in the NHS and in the private and voluntary sectors have had little exposure to people from other lands or to non-Christian faiths, and this guide intends to act as an introduction to these topics. It will also act as a reference document, to assist all personnel involved in the delivery of primary health care to offer an appropriately sensitive service to all of its patients, irrespective of their patients' backgrounds or faiths.

The guide will assist everyone working in primary care to recognise and value the differences which may be encountered when non-indigenous patients come to the surgery for registration. Other reading material, much of which has informed the compilation of this guide and which may be of interest to the reader, is listed at the back of this book. In addition, a blank page has been included at the end of each section, where notes and comments can also be written if desired.

PRIMARY CARE: PATIENTS' RIGHTS AND EXPECTATIONS

Primary health care is defined by the Declaration of Alma Ata as

> 'essential health care made universally acceptable to individuals and families in the community by means acceptable to them, through their full participation and at a cost which the community and the country can afford. It forms an integral part both of the country's health system of which it is the nucleus, and of the overall social and economic development of that community.'
>
> (World Health Organisation, 1978)

The UK Government White Paper 'The New NHS: Modern, Dependable' (SSfH, 1997) stated clearly the intention that everyone in the nation shall have

> 'fair access to health services in relation to people's needs, irrespective of geography, class, ethnicity, age or sex. For example, ensuring that black and minority ethnic groups are not disadvantaged in terms of access to service.'
>
> (Section 8, para 5.ii)

It also states that the 'renewed NHS' will deliver

> '... a personal service which is sensitive and responsive to the needs of individual patients'
>
> (Section 7, para 1)

Prior to the publication of this White Paper, 'The Patient's Charter and You' (DoH, 1996) also indicated to patients that, under the terms of the Patient's Charter (DoH, 1991), they have a right to be treated fairly, irrespective of race, religion, or colour. 'The Patient's Charter and You' is currently available in many different languages, thus enabling this information to be accessed by many non-English speaking residents of this country. Becoming aware of their rights therefore raises patients' expectations that their particular needs should at least be recognised, even if they may not yet be met immediately by individual practitioners.

THE ETHNIC COMPOSITION OF THE POPULATION OF THE UNITED KINGDOM

As we enter the third Millennium, there is no doubt that Britain is a multi-ethnic country. From the beginning of history, our shores have proved a magnet to people from other lands, many of whom settled here. Some were seeking to extend their own countries' boundaries, some were people fleeing oppression overseas, and others had land gifted to them by Royal patronage. Indeed, in past centuries, England itself used to 'own' large areas in Northern France, to say nothing of the colonies over which the country had sovereignty in the days of the British Empire. The origin of the majority of the resident population is mixed, beginning from Roman times, through the Anglo-Saxon and Viking eras, and subsequent European alliances from the Middle Ages onward.

In recent years, the ethnic composition of the population of the United Kingdom has changed. For many years, there have been pockets of inhabitants whose origins are different from the indigenous majority; for example, in the South East of England, sailors from the Indian subcontinent settled in the Medway Towns and in Thanet, and there has for some time been a Filipino community on the Romney Marshes. This picture is not unusual; along the coast in Sussex, for example, there are small but significant Somali, Arab, and Iranian populations. This picture is replicated all around the country, with large immigrant populations to be found, for example, in the port cities of Bristol, Liverpool, and Grimsby, as well as in the major conurbations like Manchester, London, Glasgow and Birmingham.

Although the historical pattern of immigration to these shores was limited in earlier times, much of it has taken place since the beginning of the 20th Century. In particular, a considerable number of people from the Caribbean were invited to the United Kingdom after the Second World War (1939–1945), to fill the British labour market (Watson, 1997; Squires, 1991; Karmi, 1996). Asian immigration also developed at that time, when men who had joined the British Armed

Forces overseas settled in Britain and subsequently sent for their families to join them here. Some years later, Asian immigrants arrived in large numbers during the 1970s. Entire communities were expelled from Uganda in the early part of that decade, from the regime of Idi Amin, and dispersed to many countries across the world, including the UK, where many of them already held the acknowledged right to British citizenship.

Although the 1991 Census indicated that the ethnic minority population of the United Kingdom was then 5.9% of the total population (at just over 3 million out of the total of approximately 55 million people) (Karmi, 1996), no question about religious affiliation was included in that Census. The census of April 2001 did subsequently include a voluntary question about participants' religions, and the results of that census are still awaited at the time of writing.

Apart from the resident immigrant population, and converts to religions other than Christianity from within the indigenous population, it is also recognised that, for example, European Community nationals, and travellers, also require regular medical attention whilst in the United Kingdom, and thus their needs must also be recognised and addressed.

In major conurbations throughout the United Kingdom, such as in Birmingham, where 13.9% of the population in 1997 was of Pakistani origin (Runnymede Trust, 1997, p.14) or Bradford, 9.5% (ibid), a Muslim patient visiting his GP, or being admitted to hospital, might reasonably expect that some of the health care professionals caring for him would be of the same faith. They might also possibly share a similar cultural background; if not, they might have easy access to information about the requirements of his religion and culture through guidelines and/or local NHS chaplaincy.

Rural communities are very different, having smaller pockets of population, and with many areas of recognised deprivation. Many GP practices in these areas may know that they have very few patients from minority ethnic groups. In some areas where there is no perceived need for this information, patients registering with a new GP may not be asked whether they have particular religious affiliations. Where practices recognise that they do have 'minority group' patients on their lists, these patients may be perceived, accurately or not, to have become 'Westernised', or less compliant with the requirements of their religion or culture, and thus therefore may not be perceived as requiring culturally sensitive care. Due to this limited exposure and, frequently, to the lack of formal specialist training provision, the situation for health care professionals may be that they have no mechanism for familiarising themselves with the particular needs of patients following differing religions and having varying ethnic origins.

Nationally within the United Kingdom, it is recognised that the needs of minority groups are an issue for consideration within the overall range of health needs of the population. Particular sensitivity needs to be fostered towards their needs. Local and national initiatives now make it clear that work is being undertaken to remove all barriers to health care, including those relating to ethnicity and religion.

REFUGEES AND ASYLUM SEEKERS

The United Kingdom's constitution is such that it recognises the needs of people from all over the world who are in fear of their lives from persecution on religious or ethnic grounds. Subject to their being able to prove their case, we have always welcomed refugees, be they for example Huguenots fleeing from France and Northern Europe, German and Polish Jews fleeing from the Nazi oppression, British Asians expelled from Uganda under the Amin regime, or Afghans fleeing the civil war in their mountainous country.

The picture began to change rapidly in recent years when simmering discord once again flared up into war in the former Yugoslavia, and Serb Christian forces began a programme of ethnic cleansing against the Albanian largely Muslim population. Thousands of people began to enter this country's sea and air ports, both by legal and illegal means. Due to Government policy at the time, the majority who claimed asylum on landing were initially housed near their ports of entry, resulting in large numbers of people being allocated accommodation in, for example, Kent and the Medway towns, as well as in the major cities with international ports and airports.

As an example of the numbers of incoming potential patients requiring health care, the then East Kent Health Authority reported that in March 2000, 3600 asylum seekers were registered with local GPs, and that approximately 25% of these were unaccompanied minors. These high numbers were undoubtedly due to the location within that part of the country of the sea ports of Dover, Folkestone and Ramsgate, with ferry services arriving from Europe daily, and the Channel Tunnel terminal at Folkestone with a Eurostar rail station some miles inland at Ashford.

It is important that the indigenous population recognises that, although economic migrants undoubtedly exist, the majority of those seeking access to asylum are fleeing oppression, torture, and religious intolerance. Many of the people who walk our streets, who the law does not permit to work whilst their cases are being considered, may be well-qualified professional people in their own countries. Both refugees (and indeed, all immigrants) and the host population need to be aware that their cultural norms, and consequently their behaviour, may be different, and misunderstandings can therefore arise.

Although this population may be transient, the NHS undertakes to offer free health care to the refugee population, both at their places of entry and at their final destinations (SSfH, 1989). In recent years, special primary care facilities have been opened up for asylum seekers. Incomers now undergo health checks before being allocated to GPs near their current places of residence.

The health care services offered by the asylum seekers' practices are delivered in such a way as to be acceptable to people from many differing ethnic and religious backgrounds, and offer interpretation facilities. This provision ensures that asylum seekers are enabled to access and use fully the local GP services, including screening.

It may be helpful to health care personnel to describe here the various recognised rights of residency under which the population of the United Kingdom is classified. The following are useful definitions:

> - **Citizens**, who have a legal right to residency in this country. Cohen states that citizenship is 'a basis for leverage within State institutions for pursuing appropriate resources for their needs';
> - **Denizens**, who have right of residency or domicile, but who have not been granted citizenship. This group may travel in and out of the country at will, and may be making considerable contributions to the country's economy;
> - **Helots**, who include illegal immigrants, and asylum seekers whose right to stay in the host country has not yet been determined. The current system for determining the right to asylum can result in some helots being resident in the UK for a number of years before their cases are considered and resolved.
>
> (Cohen, 1994)

Anyone from these groups may seek health care treatment under the NHS. Whether this is provided free of charge depends upon a number of factors, and, in primary care, these are notified to GPs through regulatory documents from the Department of Health (such as SSfH (1989)).

CULTURE AND HEALTH

Several publications have been produced in recent years about the health care needs of the immigrant population; many of these refer specifically to their requirements and preferences whilst being treated in hospital. The need for sensitive treatment of patients in the primary care setting, irrespective of their origins, is no less great. An awareness of the needs of people with differing backgrounds is essential for all primary health care professionals This has been recognised by the Government, and was referred to in the White Paper: 'The New NHS: Modern, Dependable' in 1997, and has since been reinforced with the publication of the report 'The Future of Multi-Ethnic Britain' (Parekh, 2000), which is likely to be used as a guidance document in future. Both these public documents stipulate that the training of health care professionals in cultural awareness is absolutely essential.

> 'Education – at least to the level of basic awareness – on the needs of minority groups should be an essential part of preparation for all those who plan to work in health care.'
>
> (Bahl, V., in Hopkins & Bahl, 1993)

Health care professionals will be familiar with the epidemiology of the residents of their own local area. The local demography is also known, and most health care professionals can describe their practice profile. This profile is based on the patient population and the conditions and diseases endemic to those people. Their health is affected by many factors, amongst which are income levels, housing, education, and diet.

These same factors affect everyone in the world. All patients, wherever their origins, are affected by their individual diets and personal beliefs and circumstances as well as by their cultural backgrounds and, possibly, the dietary and normative requirements of their religious practices.

People with different cultural backgrounds may also handle their illnesses differently. As an example, people from the Asian sub-continent may present with stomach pains. These pains may possibly not be gastric in origin; Asian patients are known to somatise mental stresses into digestive disorders, and these may often be treated by recognising that counselling or the ability to discuss problems openly, rather than treating the symptomatic stomach disorder, may improve the patient's general health.

It is important that the health care professional understands these factors, since a patient may present in the surgery with symptoms of illness which it is possible to diagnose wrongly if that professional is not familiar with the possible options. All primary care personnel need to be aware of the differences; we are not all the same in our presentation of illness. Language difficulties for non-English speakers, or patients for whom English is not the first language, may also make it less easy for those patients to convey how they feel, and the need for an efficient interpretation service for all patients is recognised and recommended.

A patient's cultural background has a great influence on their health. Just because an illness is traditionally treated with what might be described as 'folk medicine' does not mean that the condition could be better treated with conventional medicines. Many Eastern people believe that food and drink have 'hot' and 'cold' properties, influencing different body parts and systems, and believe therefore that eating certain foods will cure or assist specific conditions (Karseras & Hopkins, 1987). Likewise, religious practices and prohibitions must be recognised by the health care professional as being of utmost importance to the patient (Spector, 1991). 'Different' is not necessarily 'wrong' just because it is unfamiliar. A health visitor suggesting that an Asian mother should wean her baby onto proprietary foods in jars may cause consternation, when for generations the babies in that family have been weaned on naan bread and mild curries, preparing them for their preferred spicy diet in later life.

Cultural and religious issues may affect minority group patients from cradle to grave. Neile (1997, p.118) comments that 'a service is only relevant if it caters for the perceived needs of the population which is using it'. She quotes as an example the fact that a woman from an ethnic minority group may not attend antenatal classes if the information and advice given there differ from her cultural norms. Religious issues apply equally in these situations.

At the other end of life, religious communities may have particular requirements for the cleansing and disposal of the body of one of their number. As an example, Gatrad (1994) cites the difficulties which Muslim patients may face when a family member dies. Muslims prefer to die in their own homes, amongst their family and others of their faith. He describes the difficulties which Muslim families often encounter in obtaining speedy death certification, in order to comply with their religious requirement that a dead person should be buried as quickly as possible. He adds that post-mortems are not allowed within Islam; it is accepted that, in the United Kingdom, this may be demanded by the law, but this can cause further delay and distress to relatives.

The link between culture and religion is strong, and is indistinguishable in daily life in many parts of the world (Henley, 1979). Again taking Islam as an example, the behaviour of society in Muslim countries is based on teachings which cover every aspect of life and social interaction. It is often difficult for the Westerner to distinguish those aspects of behaviour which stem from religious beliefs, and those which have developed over time in people's native countries or districts. Practising Muslims will follow Islamic codes of conduct irrespective of where in the world those people originate, or where they now live. Westerners may erroneously perceive this way of life as, for example, 'Arab' or 'Pakistani', according to the origins of the person under discussion. A British Muslim woman may adapt traditional British garments to comply with the Islamic requirement for modest dressing. In the same way, people from other lands will follow religious and traditional ways of life which accommodate their individual native circumstances. The health care professional must always bear in the mind that religious and cultural norms of the immigrant and indigenous populations are equally worthy of consideration and respect.

In many ways, people entering and settling in this country have influenced British society throughout history. Lazarus (1997) points out that, latterly, immigrants have become an instrumental part of the evolution of current society. We have been introduced to a proliferation of international cuisine on our high streets, which the majority of us accept readily (McCrystal, 1996). McCrystal goes on to say that he believes that the nation is at last learning to accommodate 'things of non-white foreign origin'. However, the cultural issues and behaviours of individual minority groups may still be misunderstood, and many of the difficulties still experienced by those groups in health care matters may arise from the ignorance or uninformed prejudice of individual practitioners. Sometimes, misunderstandings can simply be resolved by discussion and explanation; intervention at an early stage can prevent expressions of anger, frustration and dissatisfaction from both health care professional and patient. For example, a patient declining to take medication presented in capsule form may not be being difficult; there may be a genuine understanding that capsules often contain gelatin, which as a pork by-product is prohibited to Jews and Muslims alike.

In comparatively recent times, vegetarians were sometimes mocked by their carnivorous fellows; it is not so very different to follow a kosher or halal diet, but these are nevertheless perceived as 'foreign' by many native British people, and treated with some suspicion. It is a point of discussion to note that the Jewish people, who number many less that the Muslim community in the United Kingdom, are generally better accepted, possibly because they tend to dress in Western styles, and do not therefore look or seem different to the onlooker (Watson, 1977).

Ineffective communication can be a barrier to effective health care. The fact that older first generation women from the Indian subcontinent rarely spoke good English continues to present considerable problems in areas such as women's health, where many women still remain unaware of the availability of screening programmes (Kubba, A., in Rawaf & Bahl, 1998). This problem is now also replicated amongst the transient refugee and asylum seeker population.

Language difficulties also arise in consultation, where much can be lost in translation, due to lack of understanding (Ahmed, T., *ibid*). Basic comprehension about the workings of the human body cannot be assumed in any patient, and limited knowledge, and differences in terminology and phrasing can lead to considerable misunderstandings. Health care professionals will be aware that when giving advice or instruction to anyone, it is essential to check verbally that these have been understood. This is particularly important in situations where the patient has a limited grasp of spoken English. It is not sufficient to ask questions which merely require 'yes' or 'no' answers, clarification must be sought as to the course of action which the patient is to take. A health visitor examining an unwell baby may ask the mother whether the baby has been sick. The health visitor intends to ask whether the baby is vomiting; 'sick' to any mother with poor English may merely mean 'unwell' and, if inaccurate terminology is being used in this conversation, inappropriate advice might then result.

In some areas, the needs of the elderly immigrant are poorly addressed; many of the elderly speak no English at all, and many find it difficult to understand that native Britons treat their old people very differently from the way that they would expect in their birth country (Admani, K., in Hopkins & Bahl, 1993). One example of potential unmet health and social care need is that elderly Asian patients are often restricted to their own homes through their inability to communicate, and many have a high incidence of rickets, due to their lack of exposure to sunlight limiting their access to naturally occurring Vitamin D. Because they remain in their homes, they do not interact with their host neighbours, and thus remain isolated within their families (Oram, 1997).

To attempt to circumvent translation difficulties, many areas of the NHS have negotiated interpretation contracts with agencies such as Language Line, under which the majority of languages can be interpreted, either as a three-way telephone conversation, or in person.

INTOLERANCE AND PREJUDICE, ASSIMILATION OR INTEGRATION?

Ahmad & Atkin (1996) comment that the United Kingdom has traditionally thought of itself as being a tolerant society. They go on to say that this view has been challenged since the 1950s, when the first waves of immigrants entered the country, brought in to work by the then Government. The Ugandan Asian influx of British citizens in the early 1970s fuelled a wave of underlying and overt racism, which has been evident from time to time as an undesirable theme ever since. This unfortunately flares up on occasion, sometimes in our major cities and frequently now also directed against the asylum seeker population. Disaffected youth amongst the minority population itself may often be involved, and immigrant groups may dispute amongst themselves; the Handsworth riots in Birmingham in the 1980s were between Asian and Afro-Caribbean peoples, at that time resentful of each others' positions in the local communities.

It may be assumed that, in order to settle down and build a life in their new country, first generation immigrants desire to be accepted by the host population whilst still retaining links with their places of origin. This desire often causes conflict. Birth country influences can be very strong, particularly when they are founded on religious practices, and there is an overwhelming desire that these should not be forgotten. Strong links often remain with their birth country, with members of their families remaining there (Watson, 1997), and extended return visits often made. Split loyalties can result, with immigrants feeling a strong need to assimilate themselves into their new community by conforming to the norms of the host country, but wishing sincerely to retain and practice the culture of the place of their birth. This need to conform, to assimilate and become like those already in the host country, is discussed by Lazarus (1997). He believes that nowadays, integration is preferable to the immigrant, rather than assimilation. He describes that, for example, the culture of the Pakistani or Arab person is so strong that, although most will accept and adhere to the law of their adoptive country, there is no way that they would wish to deny their cultural and religious origins (Joly, 1995; Constantinides, P., in Watson, 1997).

A prime example of this is the often-misunderstood practice of arranged marriages. Although forced marriages are unacceptable, the arranged marriage, when conducted properly, can be an admirable process for all concerned. The concept that both families of the intending participants are fully involved and satisfy themselves that their family backgrounds, social standing, standards and lifestyles are compatible, gives them confidence that their respective offspring will commit themselves to a union in which they will not encounter unexpected cultural demands, and which is fully supported by their families. In cultures when divorce and extra-marital relationships are unacceptable, a firm foundation is thus established from the outset. Because of the demands of the parental 'wish list', it is frequently the case that suitable marriage partners are not found within the UK population of that particular minority group, and in these instances the partner is sought in the homeland amongst family and friends still resident there.

This single example demonstrates that, in one area of life alone, the process of integration requires considerable understanding and input from the indigenous population of the host country. We need to accept that the newcomers may be different, and value them for that difference. True integration will come when the whole community can acknowledge each others' lifestyles without discomfort or embarrassment, recognise the value of diversity in the population, and embrace the way in which newcomers to our shores enrich our national culture. However, in practice, the newcomers have often been perceived as a threat to the 'British' way of life, and rather than being welcomed, they can be ignored or ostracised.

It is not surprising, therefore, that minority groups are often more comfortable with situations which are familiar to them, or where they can be assured of a certain level of sensitivity. McAvoy & Donaldson (1990) state that since the late 1950s, some 24% of doctors in the NHS have come from outside the United Kingdom, and approximately 84% of these are of Asian origin. A group of Asian GPs is likely to attract many Asian patients, particularly if they are the only such practice in a locality.

It is important that health care professionals recognise that certain ethnic groups have a predisposition to certain illnesses or medical conditions. Instances of these conditions are, for example, that diabetes and coronary heart disease are very common amongst the South Asian population (Raleigh *et al.*, 1997); genetic conditions such as sickle cell anaemia are endemic in black people with African or Afro-Caribbean origins (Chapple, J. & Anionwu, E., in Rawaf & Bahl, 1998); and thalassaemia is another condition affecting many people from Asia and Africa. The recognition of the possibility of these predispositions may assist health care professionals to diagnose previously unfamiliar conditions in their patients.

The immigration process itself may cause health problems in many people. They may find themselves alone in the host nation, and may find that they need to settle in communities which are potentially hostile, and where their customs and needs may not be understood or tolerated. In particular, the refugee community may need urgent mental health care. Many have suffered appalling levels of deprivation, or torture and fear, in their homelands or in transit, and have reached these shores under very difficult conditions. Immigration officers are not medically trained, and initial symptoms of illness may go unrecognised (Karmi, G., in Rawaf & Bahl, 1998). Some of the refugee women are pregnant, in the mistaken belief that this will advance their eligibility for housing and other benefits (Downing, 1999).

On a social level, refugees are not always welcomed by less well informed local people, since they may be perceived as a drain on local resources and funding; the refugees are often unwell due to their experiences mentioned above, and they must be allocated to already stretched GP practices. Once there, issues about the health care system may well arise; for instance, they will be unfamiliar with the processes in a system like the NHS, and thus fail to appreciate relatively simple issues like the importance of keeping to timed appointments in the surgery. In addition, language difficulties may lead to non-compliance.

To counteract these difficulties, a basic understanding amongst health care professionals of the situation of the refugee and asylum seeker population will assist them in formulating a sensitive approach to this particular patient group.

INEQUALITIES IN HEALTH

It is recognised that a large proportion of the immigrant population lives in relative deprivation. 'One-third of the officially homeless are drawn from ethnic minority groups' (East Kent Health Authority, 2000b, p.14), and 'people from minority ethnic groups are at a greater risk of violent crime and of racial harassment' (ibid, p.15). Many have little understanding of their rights to welfare benefits and services which might improve their living standards (Ahmad & Atkins, 1996). It is also noted that higher numbers of immigrants are likely to be found in areas of high population and social deprivation.

Where there is deprivation, there is poor health, irrespective of background. Economic and cultural issues, as well as ethnic and religious considerations, must be taken into account when planning services (Tovey, 2000). The 1998 report of the NHS Ethnic Health Unit recommended that strategies should be developed to meet the needs of ethnic minority patients.

Whilst planning such strategies, we must not forget that the definition of cultural differences is not exclusive to people from other countries; there are many different cultural divides between people within the United Kingdom, emanating from differences such as income, housing, education, and social class. Differences between health care professionals and their patients in perception of any situation must be set aside here if effective health care is to be delivered, and the same provision must be made for the immigrant population.

The success of local implementation of the Green Paper 'Our Healthier Nation' (SSfH, 1998), with its message of equality of access to health care for everyone, will depend on the ability of all health care professionals to deliver appropriately designed care to meet the needs of all individuals, irrespective of their origins and beliefs.

The identification (at the time of joining a GP's list) of patients from ethnic and religious minority groups may assist general practice in planning future services, and in particular in recognising potential health and special needs (SSfH, 1998).

THE RESEARCH BEHIND THE PRODUCTION OF THIS GUIDE

General medical practice is usually the first point of contact with the NHS for the majority of patients. It is frequently stated that 80% of all medical interventions take place within primary care. The White Paper 'The New NHS: Modern, Dependable' (SSfH, 1997) clearly indicated the intention that this trend will continue to develop with Government support, thus assisting to relieve the burden of care within the secondary sector.

Recent research (Timmins, 2000) investigated the ability of general practices in a large rural area, with perceived low numbers of patients from minority groups, to deliver appropriately tailored and sensitive care to any patient who might present from any one minority ethnic or religious group. This was measured by assessing the basic levels of awareness of all personnel in participating surgeries, including the GPs, about various aspects of ethnic minority cultural and religious life and their potential effects on the delivery of health care.

The results of the research revealed that, amongst the practices surveyed,

- there are a number of general medical practices, headed by GPs who are themselves from differing cultural and/or religious backgrounds, where the staff are well-informed, and to whom patients requiring recognition of, and adherence to, specific practice will gravitate;

- there are surgeries serving areas in which colleges and other nationally-recognised centres of education are situated, and where overseas students are admitted, which are well-informed and able to offer appropriate services to their patients;

- conversely, many participating practices had little or no knowledge of the needs of minority groups. They reported that they had very few or no such patients on their lists, and believed that this was an unlikely prospect. However, the future arrival of one minority group family in their catchment area, with particular needs, might mean that those needs may not be met with sensitivity, since the staff are unaware of their cultural origins and/or preferred practices, which might affect health care interventions;

- even where the awareness of individual members of staff was found to be limited, it had been expected that GPs, as independent contractors and employers within the NHS, would have access for themselves and their staff to appropriate literature and resources regarding the needs of patients of different faiths and cultures. The responses from the participating surgeries indicated that this is not always the case.

ACTION REQUIRED IN THE NATIONAL HEALTH SERVICE

It may be perceived that the National Health Service in the United Kingdom has been slow to respond in some areas to the needs of minority ethnic and religious groups, wherever their origins. The Government White Paper 'Health of the Nation' (SSfH, 1992) highlighted the importance of addressing the health needs of people from ethnic minorities. Professor Balarajan's subsequent work for the Department of Health (DoH, 1993) makes specific reference to the ethnic minority population of the United Kingdom, and to the morbidity and mortality patterns attaching to specific groups within that population. Subsequent Government documents have built upon these foundations.

Patients' perceptions of the ideal sensitive and responsive health care service may, however, be quite different in practice. Neile (1997) quotes from Weller (1991), who stated that

> '.... (the NHS) remains essentially geared to the attitudes, priorities and expectations of the majority population, which is considered white, middle class, and nominally Christian.'

More recently, Ahmed commented that

> '.... current health care provision is based upon Western medical models, which do not reflect the beliefs, values and attitudes to health held by minority ethnic communities.'
>
> (Ahmed, T., in Rawaf & Bahl, 1998)

Referring particularly to primary care, the report for 1994-97 from the Director of the NHS Ethnic Health Unit (EHU) (NHS Confederation, 1998) found that many patients from minority groups did not know that they have a right to ask for an interpreter, and that family members were often used for this service. They also found that where good practice existed, it depended upon GPs using whatever resources were available to them to enable them to provide sensitive services. The report particularly commented that

> '.... all members of the primary health care term require training. This is particularly true of front-line staff, to enable them to provide culturally sensitive care, ...and female health professionals to examine women patients.'
>
> (p. 5)

The work produced by the EHU suggested that, throughout the country, minority patient groups 'are keen to work with the NHS at all levels. Their requests for service provision are practical and modest in terms of resources'.

The EHU recommends that the following specific improvements are needed in general medical practice:

- all members of the primary health care team should have access to training in cultural and religious awareness;
- appropriate patient information should be available in foreign languages appropriate to local patients;
- female health professionals should be employed, to examine female patients;
- robust and available interpretation services should be easily accessible.

The recent research evidenced that the lessons learned by the EHU have not reflected fully into primary care in rural parts of the United Kingdom. The overall picture regarding levels of awareness of minority cultural and religious issues amongst staff in these practices can be improved. The levels of awareness identified can be described on a scale from 'highly aware and able to deliver a sensitive service' to 'not aware, and delivering a service which meets the needs of the indigenous population and is therefore assumed to meet the needs of any minority patients which we may have'.

Education and training

It is acknowledged that for clinical staff, training in cultural issues should ideally form part of their pre-qualification medical and nursing programmes (Karmi, 1996), but non-clinical staff may have very little opportunity to undertake this training. McAvoy & Donaldson (1990) recognise that

> 'there really is little point in the clinical members (of the team) enhancing their capacity to help (minority) patients, when all is undone by patient-contacts with receptionists or secretaries who have not had such training.... this is an immensely sensitive area of staff development...'
>
> (p. 36)

Individual GP practices, and the personnel who work in them, can make considerable inroads into improving access for patients from minority groups, and to improving the sensitivity of care which they receive.

The research found that many surgeries do not ask new patients whether they have any particular religious affiliations, although for many minority group patients this will form an integral part of their daily life (Henley, 1979). This is therefore an important question, which should ideally be asked at the outset. It is possible that it is raised later when treatment is necessary, but it is equally possible that it may not be considered at all, because it has never been perceived necessary. This situation might not present a problem to non-religious or non-observant patients, or to those following religions where most medications and their presentations, and medical interventions, are generally acceptable. Certain religions, however, forbid their followers from eating and drinking certain substances, and have very strong views about certain medical interventions (Karmi, 1966). Several common medications presented in capsules may be formulated with the pork by-product, gelatin, which Muslims and Jews may not consume; likewise, certain liquid medications have an alcohol base, which is forbidden by many religions. Particular care needs to be taken with the religious prohibitions of certain patients, for instance in treating diabetic patients: Hindus (to whom the cow is sacred) will not accept beef insulin, and Muslims (with a prohibition against pork) will find pigs' insulin unacceptable. Apparent cases of non-compliance with medication in these patient groups may therefore be resolved by a change of prescription to something which is acceptable to the patient. In addition, the practice of fasting on certain days must also be taken into consideration when prescribing or recommending oral medication.

It can also be significant, particularly in an emergency or in case of death, to know whether a patient requires particularly sensitive treatment on religious or cultural grounds (*ibid*).

Practices who are unaware of the cultural and religious backgrounds of their patients may run the risk of believing that cultural awareness is not relevant to them when planning health care. For instance, an opinion that the raising of cultural issues during family planning training is irrelevant to an individual surgery's practice population, presupposes that health care professionals are treating every patient the same, disregarding through lack of awareness any personal (and possibly unvoiced) needs which the patient may have. All patients may have personal or cultural preferences about contraception. Any patient, irrespective of background, who feels that they have no choice may not ask for special consideration, and many might be reticent in being outspoken about a potentially delicate subject such as this.

A presupposition that a surgery which currently has no minority group patients does not need to educate its staff in at least the basics of this important topic, is an insular view, although it is recognised that practices have to decide their individual priorities for themselves. It should however be remembered that primary care is expected to deliver a sensitive service to all patients, and it cannot be assumed that any one surgery will never have a patient from a minority group on its lists.

Practice documentation

Information available to patients may also need to be reviewed. Many surgeries already provide practice information leaflets in a wide variety of languages, but many are reliant on being sent relevant documents, and some may only provide a very limited range. Even if practices do not keep an up to date store of leaflets, it is important that they know where to obtain them, and where to access appropriate translation facilities in order to produce their own practice information documents in languages appropriate to their patient population. However, even this may not address the problem entirely. The provision of leaflets either in English or in mother tongues does presuppose that all patients are able to read; it is however known that many first-general immigrants are illiterate in their own languages, and many of the Asian languages, for instance, have very specific dialects known only in small regions of their home countries. It is therefore essential in all patient interactions to make sure that the patient, or the person providing translation, fully understands the terminology being used and the instructions and recommendations being given to the patient. Without clear communication channels, patients with a poor command of English will not experience the equality of access to NHS services which was envisioned in 'The New NHS: Modern, Dependable' (SSfH, 1997).

Consultations

Another area which needs to be considered in the improvement of the delivery of sensitive patient care is the area of the consultation itself.

Irrespective of their ethnicity or religion, many patients on a GP's list may have a preference whether they see a male or female GP. Many women, irrespective of background, prefer to see a female GP or the female practice nurses for advice on obstetric and gynaecological matters. This issue becomes very important for communities such as Muslims, where women are reluctant to expose their bodies in public to other women, and are forbidden by their religious code from exposing their bodies to men other than their husbands (Henley, 1979). The preference for single-sex consultations may apply equally to Asian men, who may additionally have a cultural aversion to being seen by a female nurse, as nursing was at one time considered a low-caste activity on the Indian sub-continent (*ibid*).

The topic of chaperon(e)s is equally important to all patients, irrespective of their origins, and should also be of significance to health care professionals themselves. There have been well-publicised recent cases where male medical practitioners have been accused of indecent assault whilst conducting examinations on their female patients; as a result, many doctors (both in primary and secondary care) now prefer to be chaperoned. In many surgeries, this option is available in primary care both to patients and staff, usually on request, in the majority of surgeries. This facility may not always be used, but it is available. Difficult situations may also arise between male patients and female practice nurses, yet the research showed that amongst the participating surgeries, only approximately 80% could offer chaperoning facilities for nurse consultations.

Offering equality of availability to services in these ways can be a problem in practices with single-sex GPs (and this applies equally to group practices and single-handed surgeries). A quarter of practices surveyed reported that a patient had declined to join their lists because only single-sex GPs were available to them. Patients are therefore disadvantaged if they are unable to consult a GP who is acceptable to them on cultural and religious grounds, and this disadvantage can be applied across the whole spectrum of patients.

Interpretation facilities

The question of interpretation continues to be an issue for practices with patients who have little or no command of the English language. Many such patients will therefore not understand even if the conversation is slow and clearly enunciated in English (Derby Conference, 2000). Many practices subscribe to translation facilities such as Language Line, but many confirm that the practice of using family members for interpretation is widespread (Henley, 1979). Care must be taken in these instances, firstly to ensure that the questions and the patient's answers are accurately translated, and secondly that possible prejudices or embarrassment on the part of the amateur translator do not affect the interpretation. On both cultural and religious grounds, it is not always seen as appropriate in certain minority groups for a husband to attend a consultation if his wife has gynaecological problems, and it is felt indelicate if a child does so. Breaches of confidentiality can also arise in the use of family interpreters (NHS Confederation, 1998).

It is not uncommon for family members to be used to interpret for indigenous patients who are deaf. The same issues arise for minority group patients, and it is not clear whether there are in fact foreign language interpreters fluent in sign language available in the NHS.

Interpretation is recognised as being an area fraught with difficulties, and although there may be no perceived language problems in some practices, there may well be unrecognised and unmet cultural norms and religious requirements due to inadequate interpretation facilities.

◆

Although many GP practices throughout the United Kingdom are undoubtedly delivering highly appropriate services, many minority group patients in areas where their population is low in number may be receiving a primary health care service which, by default, is not a 'personal service … sensitive and responsive to the needs of individual patients'. Many practices may not yet be offering the equality of access described as 'fair access to health services in relation to people's needs, irrespective of geography, class, ethnicity, age or sex'. These requirements were both outlined in the White Paper 'The New NHS: Modern, Dependable' (SSfH, 1997) as national standards for the delivery of equitable health care to the entire population of the United Kingdom.

It is hoped that this guide will be a useful tool, assisting primary health care practitioners to recognise and acknowledge the requirements of their minority group patients, and to develop and deliver appropriately sensitive services to those patients.

FORMS OF ADDRESS

Some of the more common naming systems are described under the appropriate sections of this guide. Since patients of many religious backgrounds may be registered with general practices, it will be perceived as a sensitive approach if registration forms and other documents refer to 'first' or 'given' names, rather than 'Christian' names. It is likely that the majority of people from other faith groups will understand the reasons behind the term 'Christian name' within the UK; nevertheless, the origin of the expression is clearly that this is the name with which a person is Christened, i.e. baptised into the Christian faith. To recognise diversity and to avoid any possibility of discrimination, an alternative form of reference to first or given names is desirable.

Similarly, some cultural groups may be unfamiliar with the expression 'surname', preferring the option of 'family name' (however, as will be seen later in this guide, this too can be open to misunderstanding in those cultures where several members of the same family group bear different name structures).

RELIGIOUS BELIEFS

This guide gives information about several faith groups, and about the practices and norms which followers of those faiths may wish to observe. It is important to remember that people who profess faiths may be more or less observant than the next person sharing that faith. Some people may be more relaxed about the norms and requirements of their religion than their neighbour, but their potential religious requirements must still be acknowledged.

Research in primary care revealed that general practices may have patients on their lists who are believed to follow a number of different religions, and it is those religions which are referred to in this document. It is recognised that it is not exhaustive, and the author welcomes comment from general practice staff who can identify other areas of faith and culture which should be explored and included in later editions of this guide.

It should be remembered that it is not only people from ethnic minority groups who may follow religions other than the British State faith of Christianity. There may be a perception that the indigenous population is 'White Anglo-Saxon Protestant', but this is changing. Many people of European and American origin who might be described as 'Caucasian' follow alternative religions, and faith cannot be determined – or even guessed at – by skin colour alone. The same criterion applies to people of colour, whose religious and cultural affiliations cannot be pre-assumed simply by comparing them to others of apparent similar origins.

QUESTIONS WHICH YOU MIGHT LIKE TO ASK YOURSELF PRIOR TO A CONSULTATION:

- Has the patient given me their full name?
- Do I understand the composition of the name?
- Has the patient indicated how they would like to be addressed?
- Does the paperwork in this surgery indicate 'Christian' name? If so, will this mean anything to our patients following other religions?
- Will this patient wish to have an examination by a person of the same sex?
- Will this patient wish to have a chaperon(e)?
- Will I need interpretation facilities?
- Do I understand the significance of this patient's jewellery and clothing?
- Does this patient have dietary preferences?
- Are any medications or interventions prohibited to, or disliked by, this patient? It is important to ask if I am not sure.
- Is the patient possibly fasting?
- If the patient is pregnant, is there anything special I should know about birthing arrangements?
- If the patient is dying, is there anything special I should know about their wishes?
- If the patient is bereaved, do I understand the rituals which they will wish to follow?

Most people will be pleased to be asked, and to have their dignity and wishes taken into consideration. Just because someone does not ask, it does not mean that they have no wishes – they simply may not realise that it is possible for those wishes to be realised.

THE FAITHS

1. BUDDHISM

Basic principles of the faith

Buddhism is a religion founded on the concept that people should be kind and considerate to each other, since good behaviour in this life will result in rebirth on a higher plane in the next. Buddhists believe that we should love and respect the whole of creation. Buddhists should not kill any living thing, and are expected to lead virtuous lives, avoiding stimulants such as drugs and alcohol. Self-discipline is recommended, as is open hospitality to those in need, and the giving of alms (in money or food) as a charitable deed. There is a structure of monks, who can be either men or, less commonly, women, who live simple lives and are supported wholly by the community.

Adherents to this faith follow the teachings of the Buddha, who was born in the 7th Century AD in the Nepal/northern India area, living there for some eighty years until his death. He lived simply, sharing his concepts with his followers, and concentrating on contemplation, wisdom and morality throughout his life.

The religious activities of his followers include prayers, chants, the commitment to meditation and self-awareness. The aim of reincarnation and self-understanding is that the soul will eventually reach the highest plane of consciousness, known as 'Nirvana'.

Diet

There are no religious dietary restrictions, although some Buddhists remain vegetarian, preferring to eat simply and not to wishing to consume meat products. Some Buddhists will fast regularly as a form of self-denial.

Resulting restrictions

There are no evident restrictions resulting from diet, other than an awareness that vegetarian patients may wish to avoid medication with inappropriate constituent parts.

Notes about styles of dress, jewellery, hair

There are few restrictions. Monks will shave their heads and wear saffron-coloured robes; novice monks wear dark maroon robes.

Medical interventions

The Buddhist patient recognises the sanctity of human life, and thus will accept medical care. There are no particular interventions which are forbidden to them.

Contraception and abortion

There is no specific enjoinder against contraception and abortion, particularly if the mother's life is in danger, but it may be seen to contradict the wish to preserve and value human life.

Matters surrounding birth

There are no particular restrictions relating to birth.

Matters surrounding death

Buddhists will wish to follow certain rituals at the time of death, which will vary accordingly to the sect and school of the individuals concerned. Some Buddhists believe that the body should be left for 24 hours, during which time prayers are said, and candles left burning round the room. Appropriate religious leaders will attend the body at this time. Cremation is the preferred option.

Interpreters

There are no particular difficulties noted.

Religious festivals and observances

The principal holy days for Buddhists are:

- the New Year;
- the festival simultaneously marking the birth and death of the Buddha and his elevation to the highest plane attainable, from which reincarnation will not take place.

The religious calendar is based on the lunar cycle, so the exact dates will vary from year to year. Different sects will celebrate these anniversaries on different dates.

Naming systems

The naming system is likely to relate to the patients' countries of origin.

NOTES

2. HINDUISM

Basic principles of the faith

Hinduism is a religion based on the worship of many gods, each of whom serve a different purpose. Each of these gods is believed to be a different manifestation of a single superior Being. Hinduism permeates every aspect of its followers' life – there is a considerable social and caste system inherent in the religion. They believe in reincarnation, and a person's place in the caste system in this life is consequent upon his or her performance in a previous life. The caste system also determines a person's place in the social structure, and it is rare for caste members to mix. The highest caste level is the Brahmins, who are the most devout and thus the most strict observers of their faith.

Prayer is a vital part of Hindu worship, and this takes place either in the home – every home is likely to have a shrine to their individual god(s) – or in the temple.

Diet

Hindus tend to be vegetarian, and some may not eat eggs. The cow is considered a sacred animal, and thus beef in any form is unacceptable. Alcohol and smoking are allowed, but not encouraged.

Resulting restrictions

There are no evident restrictions resulting from diet, other than an awareness that vegetarian patients may wish to avoid medication with inappropriate constituent parts, and anything containing beef extract (e.g. beef insulin for diabetic patients, beef gelatin in capsules) will be unacceptable.

Notes about styles of dress, jewellery, hair

Jewellery and religious accoutrements are important to Hindus, and they may prefer not to remove them for medical examinations. This applies to both men and women. Brahmins may wear a sacred cord around the body, and will remove it only under extreme circumstances.

Married women are identifiable by a red dot (known as a bhindi) on their forehead – this significant mark has now been adopted by some non-Hindus as a fashion statement.

Married women may also wear glass bangles on their arms. These must not be broken intentionally, because that should only be done deliberately after her husband's death.

Hindus exhort cleanliness, and, as with other religions originating in the East, believe that it is unclean to sit in washing-water, so use a shower whenever possible.

Both men and women dress modestly.

Medical interventions

There are no restrictions regarding blood transfusions or organ donation.

Traditional medicines may be used alongside NHS medications, and their use should be noted in case of interactions.

Women may not wish to expose their entire body to health care professionals, and may prefer to be examined by a female doctor or nurse.

Contraception

There are no specific instructions about contraception.

Matters surrounding birth

At birth, a holy Hindu symbol is written inside the baby's mouth using a sweet liquid.

Women prefer to remain at home for 40 days following the birth.

Matters surrounding death

Traditionally and in their homelands, deceased Hindus will be cremated on a funeral pyre, and the ashes scattered into running water. In the United Kingdom, cremation is the preferred option; many families may wish to return the deceased's ashes to their original homeland. Post-mortems are disliked.

Interpreters

Members of the elderly immigrant population may speak little or no English, but there are no particular difficulties noted.

Religious festivals and observances

The principal holy days for Hindus are

- significant birthdays of their gods, which occur throughout the year
- Diwali, the Festival of Light, when candles are lit, which occurs in the late autumn.

The religious calendar is based on the lunar cycle, so the exact dates will vary from year to year.

Every 12 years, the Khumb Mela festival takes place in northern India. Millions of devout Hindus travel from all over the world to the River Ganges to bathe, at a time in the religious calendar when it is considered that this ablution will absolve them of their sins.

Naming systems

The naming system is likely to relate to the patients' countries of origin.

NOTES

3. ISLAM

The translation of 'Islam' from the Arabic is 'submission', that is, submission to the will of God. People who follow the Islamic faith are known as Muslims (also spelt as Moslems), and they refer to God as 'Allah'.

Basic principles of the faith

Islam is one of the three Abrahamic faiths, the others being Christianity and Judaism. All three acknowledge the importance of the prophet Abraham (known to Muslims as Ibrahim). The Abrahamic faiths share many aspects and equally differ in many ways. Many of the Old Testament prophets and stories are common to all three religions.

Many people are surprised to learn that Muslims believe in Jesus (who they call Isa). They acknowledge him as a prophet, and believe that there was another prophet who followed him, who was Mohammed. The Prophet Mohammed was an ordinary man who in his fortieth year received messages through the Angel Gabriel (Jibreel), who subsequently dictated to him the holy book which Muslims follow as the Word of Allah, known as the Koran (Qu'ran).

Mohammed lived at various times in the two cities of Mecca and Medina (which are now in the modern kingdom of Saudi Arabia). These cities are the first and second holiest places in Islam. Every Muslim who has the capability to do so should visit Mecca at least once in his or her lifetime, to perform pilgrimage (known as the Hajj). In order to contain numbers attending the pilgrimage, Hajj visas are issued to enter Saudi Arabia at that time, and numbers are restricted from individual countries in the world – currently, approximately 3 million people attend Hajj every year.

Each year, the dates for Hajj to take place, and for fasting in the month of Ramadan, are determined by the Muslim calendar, which is based on the phases of the moon, and thus runs differently to the calendar widely used in the West.

The majority of Muslim patients will observe the five pillars of their faith, which are

- to make the declaration of faith, confirming that they believe that there is only one God, and that Mohammed is his Prophet
- to perform Hajj at least once in their lifetime
- to perform the five daily prayers
- to give to charity (this obligation is known as Zakat)
- to fast during the lunar month of Ramadan

The faith is based on principles of modesty, decency, cleanliness, and brotherhood. The family unit is very important, and it is relatively unusual for a Muslim male or female to remain unmarried. Arranged marriage, with the participants' consent, is frequently the norm. Sexual contact between persons who are not married is unacceptable.

Diet

Muslims are forbidden to eat pork and any pork products. They are not permitted to drink alcohol or any products containing alcohol. Some Muslims will not eat shellfish. Meat products must be 'halal', which means that the animal has been killed in the name of Allah, and that it contains no blood when prepared for the table.

During the holy month of Ramadan, the majority of Muslims will neither eat nor drink between the hours of sunrise and sunset. Many will not take any medication during the hours of fast.

Resulting restrictions

Health care professionals must be aware that their Muslim patients cannot take medication with either a porcine or an alcohol base; for example, therefore, care must be taken in prescribing insulin. Capsules containing gelatin will also be unacceptable.

Fasting is very important, and must be allowed for. If a patient is too ill to fast, they are exempted, as are menstruating women, the elderly, and pre-pubescent children – but many will wish to participate anyway.

Modesty is very important. Muslims are exhorted not to display their naked bodies (or parts of their bodies) before anyone except their marriage partners. If this must happen, consent must be sought. Most will consent to examination on medical grounds, although many may prefer to be examined by someone of their own sex.

Notes about styles of dress, jewellery, hair

Muslims are enjoined to dress modestly. For men, this means not displaying the area between the waist and the knees; for women, only the face, hands and feet should be visible. There are many cultural variations to this; strict Arab women will cover their everyday clothing from head to foot in black robes when they leave the house. Muslim women in the UK may wear a headscarf with their normal modest clothing. Many black African women will wear a colourful turban to conceal their hair.

Many Muslim men wear a beard. Other than male facial hair, bodily hair is deemed to be unhygienic, and both men and women may regularly remove all of it.

Health care professionals should be aware that some Muslims prefer to use separate towels for drying the upper and lower parts of the body. When undertaking medical examinations, the health care professional's hands should be washed before moving elsewhere on the patient's body, and separate towels used where possible.

Medical interventions

Generally speaking, the Muslim patient will welcome medical interventions; Islam encourages its followers to look after their bodily health as well as their spiritual wellbeing.

Blood transfusions are generally acceptable. Organ donation may not be so; in particular, interventions such as heart valve surgery may not be acceptable where the replacement valve is constructed from pig's tissue.

Contraception and abortion

Some Muslim patients will accept contraception, others will not. Abortion is not liked, but may be accepted on medical grounds.

Matters surrounding birth

Language difficulties have sometimes prevented pregnant immigrant Muslims accessing antenatal care. With the introduction of interpretation facilities, this should be less common.

The first words a new-born baby hears are from the Koran. Male babies will be circumcised within a few days of birth. The practice of female circumcision, which is still practised in certain parts of the world, is not an Islamic practice but originates in local culture.

Matters surrounding death

Ideally, the terminally-ill Muslim patient will wish to die at home, surrounded by his family. They will wish to hear words from the Koran read; Koranic texts are the first words heard by a new-born baby, and should be the last as the dying person departs this world.

The dead body should only be handled by fellow Muslims. The body must be washed and shrouded (ideally in the robes which the person wore when they completed the Hajj).

Muslims bury their dead, facing the direction of Mecca (south-east from the UK), ideally within 24 hours of death. Post-mortems are not liked but are usually tolerated on medical grounds.

Some Muslim families may wish to repatriate their dead to their homelands, in which case early certification of death may be requested in order to enable this to happen within the tight timescale required.

Interpreters

Many Muslims in this country are either from second- and third-generation families, and many are converts from amongst the indigenous population. There are still however a large number of people whose English is poor or non-existent (particularly the elderly). Traditionally, their children or partners have interpreted for them during medical treatment, which is not an ideal situation and can lead to prejudices and misunderstanding.

Religious festivals and observances

Muslims celebrate several holy days, the principal of which are Eid el-Fitr, which happens at the end of Ramadan, when the fast is completed, and Eid el-Adha, which takes place during the Hajj times, and reminds them of those undertaking the pilgrimage. The dates of these come forward approximately ten days every year, with the changing phases of the moon.

The Muslim holy day is Friday, when the lunchtime prayers are important.

Naming systems

The majority of Muslims will have a personal name and a religious name, e.g. Mohammed (the personal name) and Ali (the religious name). A family may not have a common surname – potentially, all the family members may have different names, although it is becoming more common that a family takes the name of the father. Married women have historically tended to retain their own names. In the same way that the Scottish 'Mac' indicates 'son of', the prefix 'bin' or 'ibn' indicates 'son of' in Muslim society.

Since the majority of Muslim patients will have a name directly related to their religion, it is often not possible to gauge their nationality from their name. Converts to Islam will adopt a Muslim name which is likely to be Arabic in origin. It is therefore important to ask a Muslim patient how they would like to be addressed.

Other useful information

Muslims follow strict rules about the use of left and right hands for certain functions. The left hand is used for washing the body after visits to the toilet, and is therefore 'unclean'; as a result, only the right hand is used for eating. They prefer to wash in running water or a shower, as the practice of sitting in dirty water during a bath is considered unclean.

After using the toilet, Muslim patients may prefer to wash their bodies with water, instead of using toilet paper. A jug, provided exclusively for this purpose, will be appreciated.

NOTES

4. JUDAISM

Basic principles of the faith

The Judaic religion is another of the three Abrahamic faiths, the others being Christianity and Islam. All three acknowledge the importance of the prophet Abraham. The Abrahamic faiths share many aspects and equally differ in many ways. Many of the Old Testament prophets and stories are common to all three religions.

The holy book of the Jews is called the Torah, which comprises the first five books of the Christian Bible, and their code of conduct is the Talmud. Their religious leaders are known as rabbis. As with Islam, Judaism affects all aspects of daily life. The most important aspects of the Torah relate to the Ten Commandments, received by Moses directly from God.

Jews in the United Kingdom are a relatively small but significant and well-established community, spread throughout the country. They follow their religion in differing ways, depending upon the sects to which they belong. Orthodox Jews are the most strict in their religious observances. Like other religions, their behaviour is based on principles of modesty, decency, cleanliness, and brotherhood. The family unit is very important. Hassidic Jews form quite a closed community, and may not mix readily with people outside their sect.

Diet

Jews are forbidden to eat pork and any pork products, and shellfish. Some Jews are not permitted to drink alcohol or any products containing alcohol. Meat products must be 'kosher', which means that the animal has been killed according to Jewish tradition.

Orthodox Jews will not eat meat and milk together, and use separate dishes and utensils for these food groups.

Jews will fast annually on the Day of Atonement – 'Yom Kippur', and may do so at other times throughout the year. Some Jews may choose to eat only cold food on a Saturday, which is their Sabbath, and on that day they are prohibited from working or carrying out strenuous activities from sunset on Friday – which can be said to include preparing meals. For Orthodox Jews, these prohibitions may also include activities such as switching on an electric light, or answering the telephone. Dietary restrictions can also apply during the holy week of Passover (Pesach), which occurs in the first quarter of the year – during this time, restrictions may apply to yeast products such as bread, cakes, and certain medications. Wine may also be replaced with unfermented wine during Passover.

Resulting restrictions

Health care professionals must be aware that their Jewish patients may not wish to take medication with a porcine base; for example, therefore, care must be taken in prescribing insulin and gelatin-based capsules. However, since the protection of life is an important aspect of their faith, this is can be waived and porcine vaccines and other medication may be acceptable – it is important to ask your patient. Your local rabbi will usually be willing to discuss individual medications and to advise which items are considered to be 'kosher', and therefore acceptable to Jewish patients.

If patients are fasting, they will not wish to take oral medication, but will accept it by other routes.

Personal modesty is important. Orthodox Jews will prefer medical examinations to be undertaken by someone of their own sex.

Notes about styles of dress, jewellery, hair

Jews dress modestly. Examples of particular requirements are:

- Orthodox Jewesses are likely to cover their hair by means of a wig, which is only removed in private.
- Hassidic Jewish men will wear their hair long in ringlets at the front, dress formally, and always wear a hat, even indoors, when away from home.
- Jewish men may frequently wear a skullcap ('yarmulke') (which is always worn in the synagogue).

Medical interventions

The Jewish patient recognises the sanctity of human life, and thus will accept medical care and certain interventions. Blood transfusions are acceptable, although organ donations may not be liked.

Contraception and abortion

Some Jewish patients will accept contraception, particularly if the mother's health is otherwise at risk. Abortion is not liked, but may be accepted on medical grounds.

Matters surrounding birth

There are no particular restrictions relating to birth.

Male babies will be circumcised, usually on the eighth day after birth. Traditionally, this duty is undertaken by a holy man known as a 'mohel'. Haemophiliac boys do not have to be circumcised, and are still considered to be Jewish without their having undergone this otherwise essential operation. Their right to be Jewish is conferred down the maternal line.

Matters surrounding death

Jewish people will be buried, preferably within 24 hours of death. The body is wrapped in a plain sheet, and someone remains with the body at all times until burial. Cremation is forbidden by Jewish law but may be acceptable. Post mortems will be discouraged unless required by law.

After the funeral, the immediate family remain at home and 'sit shivah', being visited and being brought food by relatives and friends during the mourning period, and refraining from daily activities.

Interpreters

There is a resident Jewish population for whom English is their mother tongue. Some elderly immigrant Jews may only speak Yiddish; Hebrew is the language for prayers and of more modern-day Jews. Immigrant Jews may also speak the language of their mother country. Some interpretation facilities may be required.

Religious festivals and observances

The principal holy days for Jews are

- the Sabbath (Saturdays) – from sunset on Friday until Saturday evening
- the Jewish New Year – Rosh Hashanah
- Yom Kippur – 24 hours of fasting
- Passover – in the Spring, commemorating the Exodus into Egypt
- Harvest Festival (Shavuot)
- Feast of Tabernacles (Sukkot)
- Hannukah – an eight-day festival in December, when candles are lit
- Purim, which celebrates the story of Esther

The religious calendar is based on the lunar cycle, so the exact dates will vary from year to year.

Naming systems

The majority of Jews will have names relating to their religion. The family name structure is familiar, in that wives and children take the family name of their husband and father.

The word 'ben' as part of a family name is used to indicate 'son of', as in 'David ben Gurion'.

Other useful information

The traditional Jewish diet may be high in carbohydrates, and nutrition may be inadequate.

Tay-Sachs disease has been noted as being prevalent in certain Jewish sects; this is a genetic condition of childhood which is almost always fatal.

NOTES

5. PAGANISM

Paganism is one of the oldest religions, with the belief in Mother Earth as the provider of everything, and as the main object of worship. They believe in the equality of all creation. Paganism can be found in different forms, but the central tenets are the same in the majority of them.

Since this religion can be perceived as unusual, and in some instances might appear sinister to the uninformed, Pagans may be reluctant to identify themselves unless absolutely necessary, for fear of prejudice.

Diet

Many Pagans are follow vegetarian or vegan diets, to confirm their unity with the world and all its living things. They will be reluctant to kill deliberately for food, since all creatures are seen as equals and are to be respected as such.

Medical interventions

There are no particular restrictions regarding medical or surgical interventions.

Matters surrounding birth

There are no particular birth rituals, other than general celebration of the event.

Matters surrounding death

Death is a significant rite of passage, since the soul is returning to Mother Earth. It will be important to ask the patient or family members exactly what they would like to do, both before and after death.

NOTES

6. RASTAFARIANISM

Basic principles of the faith

Rastafarianism is a social movement which established itself in Jamaica in the early 1930s. Their values combine philosophical tenets and the religious belief in a black God and Messiah. They do not, however, consider themselves as Christians.

Since Jamaica was colonised, the expression of religious belief has been one way of demonstrating resistance to oppression. Rastafarian culture combines all aspects of the slave culture and the ethics of the freedom fighters.

The name 'Rastafarian' is taken from 'Ras', meaning 'Prince', and 'Tafari', the name of the Emperor of Ethiopia, where many of the African slaves originated.

At Rastafarian prayer gatherings, 'ganja' (Marijuana) is smoked communally in a water-pipe; it is considered a holy weed.

Diet

In common with some other religions, Rastafarians will not eat shellfish or pork, or their derivatives.

Resulting restrictions

Any medication containing pork derivatives, e.g. porcine insulin, or gelatin-based capsules, will be unacceptable.

Notes about styles of dress, jewellery, hair

Many Rastafarian women dress modestly. Rastafarian men are conspicuous by their dreadlocks or long matted hair, which may be covered with a beret-type hat. The hairstyle is an important symbol of their beliefs, and should not be cut or touched without the patient's permission. Clothing colours often reflect the Rasta colours of red, green and gold.

Medical interventions

Organ transplants and blood transfusions are not generally liked.

Contraception and abortion

Traditionally, Rastafarians do not practice contraception.

Matters surrounding birth

There are no particular issues regarding birth.

Matters surrounding death

It is likely that Rastafarians will visit a dying member of their community, and may wish to pray with them.

Burial is preferred.

Interpreters

The Jamaican patois can be no more difficult to understand than other dialects. Visitors to this country may be accompanied by a local resident if interpretation is likely to be a problem.

Religious festivals and observances

All-night celebrations can be held to mark special occasions throughout the year, such as the commemoration of the emancipation from slavery, and of the anniversary of Haile Selassie I, one-time Emperor of Ethiopia.

Naming systems

The naming system is the same as that found in the United Kingdom, with a personal and family name being used.

Many people from the Caribbean will have family names which historically relate back to their slave days, in that, for instance, a slave owner named McKay would give his surname to the children born to his slaves. This family name is likely to have carried on down through the generations into the present day.

NOTES

7. SIKHISM

Basic principles of the faith

The Sikh faith developed from Hinduism in the late 16th century AD. Whereas Hindus worship many gods, Sikhs worship only one. They share many common aspects with Hindus, in particular a belief in rebirth. Their temple is known as a Gurdwara. The majority of Sikhs originated in the north-west of the Indian subcontinent.

The Sikh holy day is Sunday.

Diet

Sikhs tend to be vegetarian, although they are permitted to eat meat when the animal has been slaughtered with a single stroke. 'Halal' (Muslim) and 'kosher' (Jewish) meat is forbidden to Sikhs, although their animals are also killed in accordance with religious beliefs. Beef may be avoided, out of respect for Hindus. Pork is also considered unclean, again out of deference to Muslims. Alcohol is discouraged, but may be taken. Smoking is forbidden.

Resulting restrictions

There must be an awareness that vegetarian patients may wish to avoid medication with inappropriate constituent parts. Medicines containing beef or pork (e.g. beef or pork insulin for diabetic patients) may be unacceptable. Capsules containing gelatin may also be unacceptable.

Notes about styles of dress, jewellery, hair

Sikh men are obliged by their religion to wear the five signs of Sikhism, which are

- 'kesh' – uncut hair worn in a bun, covered with a turban
- 'kangha' – a comb
- 'kara' – a steel bangle
- 'kirpan' – a symbolic dagger
- 'kaccha' – symbolic shorts

They will be very reluctant to remove any of these symbols for any reason.

Sikh women wear their hair long, covered with a light scarf ('dupatta'). They tend to wear the traditional 'shalwar-kameez' (lightweight dress and trousers) from their homeland. Wedding jewellery is extremely important to married women.

Both men and women dress modestly.

As with other Eastern religions, Sikhs believe that it is unclean to sit in washing-water, so use a shower whenever possible.

Medical interventions

Blood transfusions and organ transplants are permitted.

Traditional medicines may be used alongside NHS medications, and their use should be noted in case of interactions.

Women may prefer to be examined by a female doctor or nurse.

Contraception and abortion

There are no specific prohibitions about contraception, although large families are considered desirable.

Abortion is allowed in extreme circumstances.

Matters surrounding birth

There are no significant requirements surrounding birth, although women may prefer to remain at home for 40 days following the birth.

Matters surrounding death

Sikh families will deal with all the death rituals of their family member. Non-Sikhs are allowed to attend the body, but the family must be consulted.

The body will be cremated within 24 hours, and the ashes scattered in running water.

Post-mortems are allowed when necessary.

Interpreters

Members of the elderly immigrant population may speak little or no English, but there are no particular difficulties noted.

Religious festivals and observances

The principal holy days for Sikhs are

- the Sikh New Year
- Diwali, the Festival of Light, when candles are lit
- a three-day holiday in early Spring
- birthdays and death anniversaries of principal figures in the faith are also commemorated.

The religious calendar is based on the lunar cycle, so the exact dates will vary from year to year.

Naming systems

It is important to understand the naming system in Sikh families.

Sikh names have three parts. The first name is personal, the second is religious, and the third is their family name.

The religious name rarely varies, and will be 'Singh' meaning a lion, for men, and 'Kaur' meaning a princess, for woman.

The family (third) name may not always be used in daily life. For example, a man's name may be (first name) Singh, or (first name) Singh (third name) – this will be the same person, and it is vital for medical records that consistency is used in recording these names.

NOTES

CHRISTIAN SECTS AND FAITH GROUPS

8. JEHOVAH'S WITNESSES

Basic principles of the faith

The Jehovah's Witnesses are Christian people, who live strictly by the teachings of the Bible. They have great respect for the sanctity of life. They believe that Jesus is the Son of God, but they do not recognise the Trinity. They use no religious symbols in worship, but believe that living a truthful life, loving one's fellow man, and demonstrating genuine love for their Maker encompass true worship. They remain neutral in hostility, yet respect authority, and do not interfere in national politics. Jehovah's Witnesses will mix freely in society, although they may not share in all recreational activities. They are probably best known for their activities in spreading the word of God (through door-to-door calling, and the 'Watchtower' publication) since they see this as a Biblical duty.

Diet

Following Biblical interpretation, Jehovah's Witnesses will not consume anything containing blood or blood products.

They believe that the Bible prohibits the use of tobacco, and addictive drugs. Alcohol is permitted, in moderation.

Resulting restrictions

The principal prohibition, arising from the Bible's instruction not to 'consume' blood, is that Jehovah's Witnesses often refuse blood transfusions. However, there is considerable discussion as to whether non-blood alternatives are acceptable, and fractions of blood may be given if acceptable to the patient. Personal choice in this matter is allowed.

It must be remembered that it is the receipt of blood which is at issue; it may be acceptable to the patient for blood to be taken for pathological analysis.

Otherwise, all medical care is sought and advice will be followed.

Hospital Liaison Committee

Jehovah's Witnesses have access to a Hospital Liaison Committee, who will negotiate with medical and nursing staff on their behalf regarding appropriate treatment involving blood and blood products. Individuals carry a small card bearing details of how the Committee can be contacted. This Committee is part of an international network, and is recognised and respected by the major institutions. The Committee will provide information for health care professionals about the Jehovah's Witnesses' views on receiving blood and blood products. It is also instrumental in making this information available to everyone through various websites on the Internet.

Notes about styles of dress, jewellery, hair

There are no particular dress habits other than modest everyday clothing appropriate to the country of origin.

Medical interventions

As stated above, blood transfusions of whole blood may be unacceptable. Individuals may decide whether or not to receive organ transplants. The extension of life by mechanical means may not be acceptable. There are no prohibitions against receiving immunisations and vaccinations.

Contraception and abortion

Contraception is permitted, abortion is not. The sanctity of life once begun must be respected.

Matters surrounding birth

There are no particular issues surrounding birth.

Matters surrounding death

Jehovah's Witnesses will wish to die naturally, and may wish to see an Elder from their community at this time. Post-mortems are acceptable, and are by personal decision. The patient's wishes may have been known in advance, and should be respected.

Interpreters

In the United Kingdom, Jehovah's Witnesses are likely to be English-speaking or, if visiting from outside the UK, they will bring an English-speaking member of their community with them to consultations.

Religious festivals and observances

Jehovah's Witnesses do not celebrate non-Christian or national holidays, nor do they recognise Christmas festivities. They will celebrate weddings and anniversaries with parties. Their only religious commemoration is that of the Memorial of Christ's death.

Naming system

This will follow that of their country of origin.

Other useful information

Jehovah's Witnesses lead morally upright lives, believing in monogamous marriage for life, with no sexual contact outside that relationship. They therefore believe that they may be protected from sexually transmitted diseases. Likewise, they believe that their standards of cleanliness may render them less likely to contract infections arising from poor hygiene habits.

NOTES

9. MORMONS

The Mormons are Christians, also known as members of the Church of the Latter-Day Saints. Their origins and main base are in Utah in the United States of America.

Mormons follow a strict moral code, and alcohol, cigarettes, and other stimulants are prohibited. At one time it was acceptable for a Mormon man to have several wives and many children, and although this practice is known to continue on occasion in outlying areas, it has been prohibited for some years.

By leading a pure life it is possible to attain the highest level of priesthood within their Church. Mormons attaining this honour will wear a ritual undergarment, which should be respected and only removed when absolutely necessary. Outer dress is otherwise modest.

NOTES

10. PLYMOUTH BRETHREN

The Plymouth Brethren are Christians, originating in Britain in the early part of the nineteenth century. They prefer simple Bible study, and their gatherings are similar to those held during Old Testament times, with hymn-singing and gospel readings. Prayers are said by the male members of the community, and they partake of bread and wine.

They are peace-loving people, and many of the original Brethren may have been conscientious objectors to military service.

Some Plymouth Brethren belong to 'exclusive' sects, that is, they like to keep themselves apart from other people. These people may wish to eat apart; they do not use computers, or listen to the radio, watch television, or read the popular press. Any such wishes should be respected. Objections to the use of computers during consultation have not been identified.

Clothing is modest and many women prefer to cover their hair with a scarf or hat.

Female patients may prefer to be examined by a female health care practitioner.

There are no restrictions applying to blood transfusions, organ transplants, and immunisations and vaccinations.

NOTES

11. THE BRUDERHOF COMMUNITY

The Bruderhof are a Christian group, with several centres in the United States of America. Their only community within the United Kingdom is situated at Nonington, outside Canterbury. The basis of their faith is following Jesus' teachings of the Sermon on the Mount, of non-violence, brotherly love, and sexual purity. They are tolerant of other faith communities.

Marriage is viewed as a unique, life-long commitment. The elderly in their community are revered. Individuals dedicate themselves to the community for life, although young people growing up are encouraged to see life for themselves in the outside world before making their own commitment. The Bruderhof believe that the common way of life provides a solution to all issues, whether political, economic or social, and they actively support the underprivileged.

They are frank people, believing that gossip is undesirable and that direct and honest address maintains open relationships and encourages friendships, since no grievances are held.

Members of the community dress modestly. The women's clothing is distinctive, often comprising a loose-fitting pinafore dress and a small headscarf worn tied at the back beneath the hair line.

In the United States, the Bruderhof run their own schools and day care centres.

Members of the community will actively seek medical advice in time of need.

The Bruderhof lead morally upright lives, believing in monogamous marriage for life, with no sexual contact outside that relationship. Single members of the community will be celibate. This may lead to a perception that they may be protected from sexually transmitted diseases and cervical cancers.

Female patients may prefer to be examined by a female health care practitioner.

NOTES

OTHER SIGNIFICANT GROUPS

12. THE CHINESE POPULATION AND CHINESE MEDICINE

Chinese people have been resident in the UK for many years, many of them having come to this country to work in the family restaurant trade. They are to be found throughout this country, and although they have integrated into mainstream life, they may often still maintain the ways of their home country in their own family and social groups.

The religion followed by the majority of Chinese is Buddhism, in several of its forms; Christianity is also followed in lesser numbers.

The Chinese naming system usually shows the family name, followed by personal name(s), although in this country many Chinese have now adopted the local style of personal name + family name. Many women follow the norm in Eastern countries of retaining their own family name when they marry.

The Chinese calendar is complex, with the months being based on a lunar and solar cycle. In order to catch up with the solar cycle, a month is added every seven years in a nineteen-year cycle. It is for this reason that the Chinese New Year falls on a different date every year.

The Chinese New Year is a long festival, commencing with the first new moon of their New Year and ending when that moon is full. The celebrations are family events, with street processions and feasts taking place; domestically, great emphasis is placed on cleaning the house, to sweep out the old year.

Many Chinese people use traditional Chinese medicines, and practitioners can be found in many towns and cities. The use of traditional Chinese medicines is now also becoming increasingly popular in some areas amongst the indigenous population. The principles behind the practice of Chinese medicine are that healthiness is subject to opposing forces within the body, which must be balanced in order to maintain good health. The use of acupuncture and appropriate medicinal treatment can release blockages in the flow of vital energy, and thus restore balance.

As with other forms of natural medicine, it is important to ascertain whether alternative medicines are being taken, in case of interactions or contra-indications when taken with prescription medicines. Strict adherence to quantities and proportions of ingredients are very important, as some of the substances used can be toxic when administered incorrectly. Health care professionals should note that the Medicines Control Agency has recently expressed considerable concerns about the regulation of the quality of products used in the formulation of Chinese medicines, and recommend that patients should ensure that a clear list of ingredients, in English, is shown on the products. Prosecutions have taken place where the ingredients have been illegal in the UK or are of low quality, presenting a potential risk to health.

NOTES

13. THE ROMA (ROMANY) PEOPLE/ TRAVELLERS/GYPSIES

Background

The travelling population is known by many names in different parts of the world. Their origins are very ancient, certainly stemming from as early as the Middle Ages. It is possible that the name 'gypsy' arose from a rumour that they came from Egypt, but it seems more likely that their origins were in northern India around the 10th century AD. The language which is common to the majority of them (Romanes) certainly contains words which have similarities both to Indian sub-continental tongues and to Arabic.

The Roma's first recorded contact with Europeans was in the 1300s. They travelled to and remained within many European countries, including Germany and Czechoslovakia, and the Irish Travellers (many of whom can be found within the United Kingdom to this day) have their origins amongst these peoples.

There is an extensive clan system which embraces all Roma families. The family unit is very important, and there is a highly defined social structure. Many Roma travel for most of the year but remain camped in one place over the winter months. They recognise the significance of interaction with non-Romanies, but intermarriage is not encouraged.

Since the Roma are used to a travelling lifestyle, there may be considerable reluctance to attend for medical treatment, and a stay in hospital may be treated with great suspicion. If a female Roma patient consents to examination, a female health care practitioner will be desirable. The Roma may find it difficult to comply with the system of appointments for medical treatment, preferring to turn up when they are willing to accept treatment. Call and recall will probably not be practical, since they are likely to have moved on. Notwithstanding these problems in integrating them into the health care system, the Roma people say that their way of life has enabled them to survive through great hardships and plagues over the centuries.

Self-diagnosis and treatment, or reference to a wise woman, are the preferred methods of health care. The Roma people make extensive use of herbal and alternative medicines. Rituals and traditions are very important to them, and certain objects, people and creatures are believed to be tainted. There is a strong belief in 'bad luck', and any such portents will be avoided.

Despite their wandering lifestyle, cleanliness and personal hygiene are held to be important, and substances such as menstrual fluids are held to be unclean.

The travelling lifestyle does however bring its own problems. Access to health care can be difficult, as there is no fixed address. If they do stay in any place for a time, allocations to GP surgeries can be unsatisfactory, since these patients may move on before diagnosis or during treatment. This moving on may be involuntary, or by their own decision.

Literacy, and the ability therefore to read and understand the written word, may present a problem in this group of patients. It is believed that more than 50% of the adult travelling population may be illiterate. Children's schooling is patchy, where they can access school places, and often fragmented by moving on.

Pregnant women rarely access antenatal care, and this may cause problems. Many women subsequently find that their medical condition or that of their unborn children is such that, due to their lack of prenatal checks, they have to undergo Caesarean deliveries, which would not be their method of choice. The women traditionally prefer that childbirth is natural and managed by other women within the family.

It is reported that traveller children are more frequently injured as a result of road accidents that the resident population, since they are more exposed to the hazards of traffic. In the case of accident, travellers will often report direct to their local A&E department.

The travelling population has a high incidence of respiratory disease.

There is also a high incidence of congenital abnormalities. Much of this may be attributed to travelling families' preference for intermarrying within the clan; similar circumstances often arise amongst families from the Indian subcontinent, where spouses are sought within the wider family group.

The Irish travelling population (sometimes referred to as 'tinkers') has the same ancestral origins as the groups currently found throughout Europe, and European Roma can still be found as a distinct group in Ireland. Both Irish and European travellers will be found at sites located throughout the United Kingdom. They are an ancient people, and remain considerably disadvantaged on all fronts in all aspects of society.

NOTES

NOTES

NOTES

NOTES

REFERENCES

This guide has been compiled with reference to the following documents, and the assistance of the respective authors is gratefully acknowledged:

Abigail, S. (2000) Plymouth Brethren, FAQs. Website accessed 31-01-2001: www.storm.ca/~sabigail/faqs/brethren.

Ahmad, W.I.U. & Atkin, K. (eds) (1996) 'Race' and Community Care', Buckingham, Open University Press.

Anaokar, M. (2000) Series of articles on religious beliefs and health care. Practice Manager Journal.

Barry, J. & Kirke, P. (1997) 'Congenital Abnormalities in the Irish Traveller Community'. Irish Medical Journal, Vol. 90, no. 6, October 1997.

Bath Health Promotion Unit (1996) 'Respect for Privacy, Dignity, and Religious and Cultural Beliefs', Bath, Bath HPU.

Bennion, Rachel (2000) 'Handbook on Cultural, Spiritual & Religious Beliefs', South Devon Healthcare NHS Trust. Website accessed 30-5-2001: www.sdhl.nhs.uk/documents/cultural.

Bradford Community Health (1999) 'Ethnic Minorities Health', vol. 10, Part 4, September .

British Broadcasting Corporation (1998) 'Burying Muslims', Transcript from BBC World Service (Religion) broadcast, January 16 1998 (London, BBC).

The Bruderhof Communities (2001) Website accessed 29-5-2001: www.bruderhof.org.

Burke, M. (1999) 'The Travellers – Ireland's Ethnic Minority'. Website accessed 10-7-2001: www.qub.ac.uk/english/~/travellers.htm.

Burnett, A. (1999) 'Guidelines for Healthworkers providing Care for Kosovan Refugees', in 'Ethnic Minorities Health', Bradford Community Health, vol. 10, part 4, September 1999.

Consumer Health Interactive & OneBody, Inc. (1998) 'Traditional Chinese Medicine'. Website accessed 29-05-2001: www.ahealthyme.com/article/primer/10026128.

Department of Health (1991) 'The Patient's Charter', London, DoH.

Department of Health (1993) 'Ethnicity and Health', a Guide for the NHS, London, DoH.

Department of Health (1996) 'The Patient's Charter and You', London, DoH.

Diabetes Training Centre (1999) 'Ethnic Minorities' module forming part of the Diploma-Level clinical training programmes in the Management of Coronary Heart Disease and Diabetes in Primary Care, Bradford, Diabetes Training Centre.

Dover Express (1999, 2000) Various articles relating to provision of services for refugees and asylum seekers.

Downing, M.H. (1999) 'Primary Health Care for Asylum Seekers in Dover and the Impact of Asylum Seekers on the Local Community', unpublished report for Channel Primary Care Group.

East Kent Health Authority (1999) 'Health Improvement Programme 2000–2003', Dover, EKHA.

East Sussex, Brighton & Hove Health Authority (2000) 'Quality Matters in General Practice', Annual Report by the Director of Public Health, Lewes, ESBHHA.

Edwards, Roanne (1999) 'Rastafarians'. Website accessed 31-01-2001: www.africana.com/tt_010.

FortuneCity (2001) 'The Romany Culture & Language'. Website accessed 31-01-2001: http://westwood.fortunecity.com/armani/208/romany.

Gatrad, A.R. (1994) 'Muslim Customs surrounding Death, Bereavement, Post-Mortem Examinations and Organ Transplants', British Medical Journal, vol. 309, 20–27 August 1994, pp. 521–523.

Henley, A. (1979) 'Asian Patients in Hospital and at Home', Tunbridge Wells, Pitman Medical Publishing Co. Ltd.

Hill, S. (1999) 'A Sensitive Approach to Issues of Ethnicity', Practice Nurse, vol. 17, no. 5, pp. 296–300.

Hinnells, J.R. (1984) 'A Handbook of Living Religions', Harmondsworth, Penguin Books Ltd.

Hopkins, A. & Bahl, V. (1993) 'Access to Health Care for People from Black and Ethnic Minorities', London, Royal College of Physicians.

Jarvis, S. (1997) 'The Pros and Cons of using a Chaperone', Doctor Journal, 16 October 1997.

Karmi, G. (1996) 'The Ethnic Health Handbook', Oxford, Blackwell Science Ltd.

Language Line (undated leaflet) 'Your 'Point Card' for Non-English Speakers', London, Language Line.

London Evening Standard (2002) 'Call for tighter law on Chinese Medicine Trade', 1 March 2002, p. 18.

Lothian Racial Equality Council (1992) 'Religions and Cultures – a guide to patients' beliefs and customs for health service staff', Edinburgh, Lothian REC.

McAvoy, B.R. & Donaldson, L.J. (eds) (1990) 'Health Care for Asians', Oxford, Oxford University Press.

Mares, P., Henley, A. & Baxter, C. (1985) 'Health Care in Multiracial Britain', Cambridge, Health Education Council & National Extension College Trust Ltd.

Ministry of Defence. Reference document for military personnel and local communities: 'The Gurkhas' (unreferenced).

Narayanasamy, A. (2001) 'Spiritual Care: a practical guide for nurses and health care practitioners', Trowbridge, Cromwell Press.

National Association of Health Authorities & Trusts (1996) 'Spiritual Care in the NHS', Birmingham, NAHAT.

National Health Service Confederation (1998) 'Composite Directory of NHS Ethnic Health Unit Projects', London, NHS Confederation.

Neile, E. (1997) 'Control for Black and Ethnic Minority Women: a Meaningless Pursuit', published in 'Reflections on Midwifery'. Kirkham, M.J. & Perkins, E.R. (eds) 1997, London, Balliere Tindall.

Oram, J.J. (1997) 'Caring for the Fourth Age', London, Armelle Press.

PageWise, Inc. (2001) 'Irish Travellers, Ireland's Minority Culture'. Website accessed 10-7-2001: mi.essortement.com/irishtravellers_ryjv.htm.

Parekh, B. (2000) The Parekh Report: 'The Future of Multi-Ethnic Britain', London, Profile Books.

Pavee Point Travellers' Centre (2001) 'Irish Travellers'. Website accessed 10-7-2001: www.iol.ie/~pavee/Travellers.htm.

Raleigh, V.S., Kiri, V. & Balarajan, R. (1997) 'Variations in Mortality from Diabetes Mellitus, Hypertension, and Renal Disease in England and Wales by Country of Birth', Health Trends, 28, pp. 122–127.

Rao, J. & Ramalah, S. (2000) 'Lip Service', Health Service Journal, 6 April 2000, p. 30.

Rawaf, S. & Bahl, V. (eds) (1998) 'Assessing Health Needs of People from Ethnic Minority Groups', London, Royal College of Physicians & The Faculty of Public Health Medicine, pp. 324 and 326.

Roche, M. & van Berkel, R. (1997) 'European Citizenship and Social Exclusion', Aldershot, Ashgate Publishing Ltd.

Sales Online Direct, Inc. (2001) 'Irish Travellers'. Website accessed 10-7-2001: www.irishclans.com/articles/travellers.html.

Secretary of State for Health (1989) 'The National Health Service (Charges to Overseas Visitors) Regulations, 1989' – Statutory Instrument 1989 no. 306, London, HMSO.

Secretary of State for Health (1992) 'The Health of the Nation', London, HMSO.

Secretary of State for Health (1997) 'The New NHS: Modern, Dependable', London, HMSO.

Secretary of State for Health (1998) Green Paper: 'Our Healthier Nation: a Contract for Health', London, HMSO.

Segal, E.L. (1995) 'The Great Passover Raisin-Wine Controversy'. Website accessed 10-7-2001: www.ucalgary.ca/~/Raisin_Wine.html.

Spector, R.E. (1991) 'Cultural Diversity in Health & Illness', East Norwalk, Connecticut, Appleton & Lange, pp. 137–142.

Squires, A.J. (ed) (1991) 'Multicultural Health Care and Rehabilitation of Older People', London, Balliere Tindall.

Timmins, S. (2000) 'Sensitive and Responsive…?' (an investigation into the ability of general medical practice in East Kent to deliver primary health care which is appropriately sensitive to the needs of minority ethnic and religious patient groups), dissertation for MSc Interprofessional Health & Community Studies award at Canterbury Christ Church University College (unpublished).

Tovey, P. (ed.) (2000) 'Contemporary Primary Care – the Challenges of Change', Buckingham, Open University Press.

University of California (2001) 'Chinese New Year'. Website accessed 10-7-2001: www.educ.uvic.ca/~/chinese_new_year.html.

Watch Tower Bible & Tract Society of Pennsylvania (2001) 'Jehovah's Witnesses'. Website accessed 30-5-2001: www,jw-media.org.

Watson, J.L. (ed.) (1977) 'Between Two Cultures: Migrants and Minorities in Britain', Oxford, Blackwell.

Weller, B. (1991) 'Nursing in a Multicultural World', Nursing Standard 5(30), pp. 31–32 (in Neile, E. (1997)).

World Health Organisations (1978) 'Declaration of Alma Ata', International Conference on Primary Health Care, Alma Ata, USSR, 6-12 Dec 1978. Website accessed 18-6-2000: www.who.dk/almaata.htm.

Extracts from author's personal notes (2000) 'Promoting Race Equality in Rural Areas' conference, Derby, 10.7.00.

Author's notes (2001) from discussion with Kent County Council's Traveller Education Welfare officer, 11.7.01.